My Sleeve Journey

My Medical History

Current Contact Info for Physicians

Insurance Information

Insurance Requirements for Surgery

List of Current Medications

Questions for Surgeon

Dates for Future Medical Visits

Dates for Nutritionist Visits

Dates for Follow Up Visits with PCP

Before Picture & Current Weight/Measurements

Questions for Doctor

Notes

Month One Pre-Op Plan

Month One: Activity Goals

General Shopping List

Thoughts about My Journey So Far

Month One Results

Non-Scale Victories (NSV)

Month Two: Picture & Current Weight/Measurements

Questions for Doctor

Notes

Month Two Pre-Op Plan

Month Two: Activity Goals

General Shopping List

Thoughts about My Journey So Far

Month Two Results

Non-Scale Victories (NSV)

Month Three: Picture & Current Weight/Measurements

Questions for Doctor

Notes

Month Three Pre-Op Plan

Month Three: Activity Goals

General Shopping List

Thoughts about My Journey So Far

Month Three Results

Non-Scale Victories (NSV)

Month Four: Picture & Current Weight/Measurements

Questions for Doctor

Notes

Month Four Pre-Op Plan

Month Four: Activity Goals

General Shopping List

Thoughts about My Journey So Far

Month Four Results

Non-Scale Victories (NSV)

Month Five: Picture & Current Weight/Measurements

Questions for Doctor

Notes

Month Five Pre-Op Plan

Month Five: Activity Goals

General Shopping List

Thoughts about My Journey So Far

Month Five Results

Non-Scale Victories (NSV)

Month Six: Picture & Current Weight/Measurements

Questions for Doctor

Notes

Month Six Pre-Op Plan

Month Six: Activity Goals

General Shopping List

Thoughts about My Journey So Far

Non-Scale Victories (NSV)

Month Six Results

Waiting on Insurance Approval (Notes)

Questions for Surgeons Office

Pre-Op Picture, Weight & Measurements

Questions for Doctor

Notes

Meeting with Nutritionist or Nutrition Class Notes

Notes

Notes

List of Items to Bring to the Hospital

Plan for Surgery Day

List of Medications

Plan for Medical Leave

Plan for Surgery Recovery

Questions for Surgeon

Notes

Dates for Future Medical Visits

Dates for Nutritionist Visits

Dates for Follow Up Visits with PCP

Directions for Pre-Surgery Diet Plan

Notes

Shopping List for Pre-Surgery and Post Surgery Diet

Week 1, Day 1: Surgery Day!!! Notes

Week 1, Day 2: Notes, Pain/Discomfort Level, Liquids

Week 1, Day 3: Notes, Pain/Discomfort Level, Liquids

Week 1, Day 4: Notes, Pain/Discomfort Level, Liquids

Week 1, Day 5: Notes, Pain/Discomfort Level, Liquids

Week 1, Day 6: Notes, Pain/Discomfort Level, Liquids

Week 1, Day 7: Notes, Pain/Discomfort Level, Liquids

Non-Scale Victories (NSV)

Measurements and Weight

Questions to Ask Surgeon

Follow Up Appointment with Surgeon (Notes)

Goals until 3-month Appointment

Activity Goals Month 1

Current List of Medications

Shopping List

Week 2: Pain/Discomfort/Periods/BM

Shopping List

Weekly Meal Planning

When I Eat Out I Eat...

Foods I Can Tolerate

Foods I Cannot Tolerate

Week 2, Weekly Meal Planning

Week 2, Water and Vitamin Goals

Week 2, Food Log, Day 1

Week 2, Food Log, Day 2

Week 2, Food Log, Day 3

Week 2, Food Log, Day 4

Week 2, Food Log, Day 5

Week 2, Food Log, Day 6

Week 2, Food Log, Day 7

Week 2, Non-Scale Victories (NSV)

Week 2, Measurements and Weight

Week 3: Pain/Discomfort/Periods/BM

Shopping List

Weekly Meal Planning

Water and Vitamin Goals

Week 3, Food Log, Day 1

Week 3, Food Log, Day 2

Week 3, Food Log, Day 3

Week 3, Food Log, Day 4

Week 3, Food Log, Day 5

Week 3, Food Log, Day 6

Week 3, Food Log, Day 7

Week 3, Non-Scale Victories (NSV)

Week 3, Measurements and Weight

Week 4: Pain/Discomfort/Periods/BM

Shopping List

Weekly Meal Planning

Water and Vitamin Goals

Week 4, Food Log, Day 1

Week 4, Food Log, Day 2

Week 4, Food Log, Day 3

Week 4, Food Log, Day 4

Week 4, Food Log, Day 5

Week 4, Food Log, Day 6

Week 4, Food Log, Day 7

Week 4, Non-Scale Victories (NSV)

Week 4, Picture, Weight & Measurements

List of Current Medications

Activity Goals, Month 2

When I Eat Out, I Eat...

Foods I Can Eat

Foods I Can't Eat

Week 5: Pain/Discomfort/Periods/BM

Shopping List

Weekly Meal Planning

Water and Vitamin Goals

Week 5, Food Log, Day 1

Week 5, Food Log, Day 2

Week 5, Food Log, Day 3

Week 5, Food Log, Day 4

Week 5, Food Log, Day 5

Week 5, Food Log, Day 6

Week 5, Food Log, Day 7

Week 5, Non-Scale Victories (NSV)

Week 5, Measurements and Weight

Week 6: Pain/Discomfort/Periods/BM

Shopping List

Weekly Meal Planning

Water and Vitamin Goals

Week 6, Food Log, Day 1

Week 6, Food Log, Day 2

Week 6, Food Log, Day 3

Week 6, Food Log, Day 4

Week 6, Food Log, Day 5

Week 6, Food Log, Day 6

Week 6, Food Log, Day 7

Week 6, Non-Scale Victories (NSV)

Week 6, Measurements and Weight

Week 7: Pain/Discomfort/Periods/BM

Shopping List

Weekly Meal Planning

Water and Vitamin Goals/Notes

Week 7, Food Log, Day 1

Week 7, Food Log, Day 2

Week 7, Food Log, Day 3

Week 7. Food Log, Day 4

Week 7, Food Log, Day 5

Week 7, Food Log, Day 6

Week 7, Food Log, Day 7

Week 7, Non-Scale Victories (NSV)

Week 7, Measurements & Weight

Week 8: Pain/Discomfort/Periods/BM

Shopping List

Weekly Meal Planning

Water and Vitamin Goals/Notes

Week 8, Food Log, Day 1

Week 8, Food Log, Day 2

Week 8, Food Log, Day 3

Week 8 Food Log, Day 4

Week 8, Food Log, Day 5

Week 8, Food Log, Day 6

Week 8, Food Log, Day 7

Week 8, Non-Scale Victories (NSV)

Week 8, Picture, Weight & Measurements

List of Current Medications

Activity Goals, Month 3

Week 9: Pain/Discomfort/Periods/BM

Shopping List

When I Eat Out, I Eat...

Foods I Can Eat

Foods I Can't Eat

Weekly Meal Planning

Water and Vitamin Goals/Notes

Week 9, Food Log, Day 1

Week 9, Food Log, Day 2

Week 9, Food Log, Day 3

Week 9, Food Log, Day 4

Week 9, Food Log, Day 5

Week 9, Food Log, Day 6

Week 9, Food Log, Day 7

Week 9, Non-Scale Victories (NSV)

Week 9, Measurements and Weight

Week 10: Pain/Discomfort/Periods/BM

Shopping List

Weekly Meal Planning

Water and Vitamin Goals/Notes

Week 10, Food Log, Day 1

Week 10, Food Log, Day 2

Week 10, Food Log, Day 3

Week 10, Food Log, Day 4

Week 10, Food Log, Day 5

Week 10, Food Log, Day 6

Week 10, Food Log, Day 7

Week 10, Non-Scale Victories (NSV)

Week 10, Measurements and Weight

Week 11: Pain/Discomfort/Periods/BM

Shopping List

Weekly Meal Planning

Water and Vitamin Goals/Notes

Week 11, Food Log, Day 1

Week 11, Food Log, Day 2

Week 11, Food Log, Day 3

Week 11, Food Log, Day 4

Week 11, Food Log, Day 5

Week 11, Food Log, Day 6

Week 11, Food Log, Day 7

Week 11, Non-Scale Victories (NSV)

Week 11, Measurements & Weight

Week 12: Pain/Discomfort/Periods/BM

Shopping List

Weekly Meal Planning

Water and Vitamin Goals/Notes

Week 12, Food Log, Day 1

Week 12, Food Log, Day 2

Week 12, Food Log, Day 3

Week 12, Food Log, Day 4

Week 12, Food Log, Day 5

Week 12, Food Log, Day 6

Week 12, Food Log, Day 7

Week 12, Non-Scale Victories (NSV)

Month 3 Picture, Weight & Measurements

Activity Goals, Month 4

List of Current Medications

Three Month Appointment (Notes)

Goals for Months 4-6

When I Eat Out, I Eat...

Foods I Can Do

Foods I Can't Do

Week 13: Pain/Discomfort/Periods/BM

Shopping List

Weekly Meal Planning

Water and Vitamin Goals/Notes

Week 13, Food Log, Day 1

Week 13, Food Log, Day 2

Week 13, Food Log, Day 3

Week 13, Food Log, Day 4

Week 13, Food Log, Day 5

Week 13, Food Log, Day 6

Week 13, Food Log, Day 7

Week 13, Non-Scale Victories (NSV)

Week 13, Measurements and Weight

Week 14: Pain/Discomfort/Periods/BM

Shopping List

Weekly Meal Planning

Water and Vitamin Goals/Notes

Week 14, Food Log, Day 1

Week 14, Food Log, Day 2

Week 14, Food Log, Day 3

Week 14, Food Log, Day 4

Week 14, Food Log, Day 5

Week 14, Food Log, Day 6

Week 14, Food Log, Day 7

Week 14 Non-Scale Victories (NSV)

Week 14, Measurements & Weight

Week 15: Pain/Discomfort/Periods/BM

Shopping List

Weekly Meal Planning

Water and Vitamin Goals/Notes

Week 15, Food Log, Day 1

Week 15, Food Log, Day 2

Week 15, Food Log, Day 3

Week 15, Food Log, Day 4

Week 15, Food Log, Day 5

Week 15, Food Log, Day 6

Week 15, Food Log, Day 7

Week 15, Non-Scale Victories (NSV)

Week 15, Measurements and Weight

Week 16: Pain/Discomfort/Periods/BM

Shopping List

Weekly Meal Planning

Water and Vitamin Goals/Notes

Week 16, Food Log, Day 1

Week 16, Food Log, Day 2

Week 16, Food Log, Day 3

Week 16, Food Log, Day 4

Week 16, Food Log, Day 5

Week 16, Food Log, Day 6

Week 16, Food Log, Day 7

Week 16 Non-Scale Victories (NSV)

Month 4 Picture, Weight & Measurements

Activity Goals, Month 5

Week 17: Pain/Discomfort/Periods/BM

Shopping List

When I Go Out To Eat, I Eat...

Foods I Can Do

Foods I Can't Do

Weekly Meal Planning

Water and Vitamin Goals/Notes

Week 17, Food Log, Day 1

Week 17, Food Log, Day 2

Week 17, Food Log, Day 3

Week 17, Food Log, Day 4

Week 17, Food Log, Day 5

Week 17, Food Log, Day 6

Week 17, Food Log, Day 7

Week 17, Non-Scale Victories (NSV)

Week 17, Measurements and Weight

Week 18: Pain/Discomfort/Periods/BM

Shopping List

Weekly Meal Planning

Water and Vitamin Goals/Notes

Week 18 Food Log, Day 1

Week 18, Food Log, Day 2

Week 18, Food Log, Day 3

Week 18, Food Log, Day 4

Week 18, Food Log, Day 5

Week 18, Food Log, Day 6

Week 18, Food Log, Day 7

Week 18, Non-Scale Victories (NSV)

Week 18, Measurements and Weight

Week 19: Pain/Discomfort/Periods/BM

Shopping List

Weekly Meal Planning

Water and Vitamin Goals/Notes

Week 19, Food Log, Day 1

Week 19, Food Log, Day 2

Week 19, Food Log, Day 3

Week 19, Food Log, Day 4

Week 19, Food Log, Day 5

Week 19, Food Log, Day 6

Week 19, Food Log, Day 7

Week 19, Non-Scale Victories (NSV)

Week 19, Measurements and Weight

Week 20: Pain/Discomfort/Periods/BM

Shopping List

Weekly Meal Planning

Water and Vitamin Goals/Notes

Week 20, Food Log, Day 1

Week 20, Food Log, Day 2

Week 20, Food Log, Day 3

# Week 20, Food Log, Day 4

Week 20, Food Log, Day 5

Week 20, Food Log, Day 6

Week 20, Food Log, Day 7

Week 20, Non-Scale Victories (NSV)

Week 20, Picture, Weight and Measurements

Activity Goals, Month 6

Week 21: Pain/Discomfort/Periods/BM

When I Go Out to Eat, I Eat...

Foods I Can Do

Foods I Can't Do

Shopping List

Weekly Meal Planning

Water and Vitamin Goals/Notes

Week 21, Food Log, Day 1

Week 21, Food Log, Day 2

Week 21, Food Log, Day 3

Week 21, Food Log, Day 4

Week 21, Food Log, Day 5

Week 21, Food Log, Day 6

Week 21, Food Log, Day 7

Week 21, Non-Scale Victories (NSV)

Week 21, Measurements and Weight

Week 22: Pain/Discomfort/Periods/BM

Shopping List

Weekly Meal Planning

Water and Vitamin Goals/Notes

Week 22, Food Log, Day 1

Week 22, Food Log, Day 2

Week 22, Food Log, Day 3

Week 22, Food Log, Day 4

Week 22, Food Log, Day 5

Week 22, Food Log, Day 6

Week 22, Food Log, Day 7

Week 22, Non-Scale Victories (NSV)

Week 22, Measurements and Weight

Week 23: Pain/Discomfort/Periods/BM

Shopping List

Weekly Meal Planning

Water and Vitamin Goals/Notes

Week 23, Food Log, Day 1

Week 23, Food Log, Day 2

Week 23, Food Log, Day 3

Week 23, Food Log, Day 4

Week 23, Food Log, Day 5

Week 23, Food Log, Day 6

Week 23, Food Log, Day 7

Week 23, Non-Scale Victories (NSV)

Week 23 Measurements and Weight

Week 24: Pain/Discomfort/Periods/BM

Shopping List

Weekly Meal Planning

Water and Vitamin Goals/Notes

Week 24, Food Log, Day 1

Week 24, Food Log, Day 2

Week 24, Food Log, Day 3

Week 24, Food Log, Day 4

Week 24, Food Log, Day 5

Week 24, Food Log, Day 6

Week 24, Food Log, Day 7

Week 24, Non-Scale Victories (NSV)

6 Month Pictures, Measurements and Weight

List of Current Medications

Questions for Surgeon

6 Month Appointment (Notes)

Goals for month 7-12

Foods I Can Do

Foods I Can't Do

Notes

Notes

Notes

Notes

Notes

Notes

Notes

Notes

Notes

Notes

Notes

Notes

Notes

Made in the USA
Coppell, TX
27 April 2023